FROM MANAGING TO CONQUERING COLON POLYPS

Expert Guide To Colon Polyps Causes, Symptoms, Treatment, And Achieving Complete Wellness

DR. DASHIELL DANIEL

CHAPTER ONE   17

COLON POLYPS   17

CHAPTER TWO   22

MEDICAL DIAGNOSIS AND TREATMENT   22

CHAPTER THREE   26

CHANGES IN LIFESTYLE   26

CHAPTER FOUR   31

MANAGING STRESS AND MENTAL HEALTH   31

Colon Polyps: A Comprehensive Guide" is a priceless tool for researchers, medical professionals, and anyone looking to learn everything there is to know about colon health and, in particular, colon polyps. This book explores many aspects of colon health and provides information on the complexity of colon polyps and how important it is to keep your colon healthy.

The first chapter establishes the framework for the remaining chapters, explaining the goal of the book and stressing the critical importance of colon health. It also defines the book's scope and emphasizes the importance of understanding colon polyps, a topic that is frequently undervalued in public discourse.

The central section of the book, "Colon Polyps 101," offers a thorough examination of the definition, kinds, causes, and symptoms of colon polyps.

The focus on early discovery highlights the need and urgency of taking preventative action in the management of this medical condition.

The following chapters—which address medical diagnosis and treatment, lifestyle changes, stress management, and prevention strategies—offer a comprehensive strategy for managing colon polyps. The book's academic rigor is enhanced by the thorough analysis of screening protocols, interpretation of test results, and variety of treatment options.

Chapter 6's real-life stories give the academic discourse a human face and a relatable dimension; patient experiences, success stories, and challenges and triumphs enhance the narrative and make the material more approachable and interesting for a wide range of readers.

The book's relevancy is further enhanced by Chapter 7's forward-looking view on future trends and research, which highlights the author's dedication to remaining up to date with new medical developments, technological advancements, and exciting research topics.

All things considered, "Colon Polyps: A Comprehensive Guide" is a landmark work that not only synthesizes prior research but also opens up new avenues for future investigation and comprehension of colon health. Its scholarly tone, along with a compelling mix of personal accounts and cutting edge perspectives, makes it an invaluable resource for researchers, physicians, and anyone interested in proactive management of colon health.

Overview

Maintaining optimal colon health is crucial for preventing various digestive disorders, and one of the major concerns in this regard is the presence of colon polyps. This discussion delves into the nuances of conquering colon polyps, exploring the importance of colon health and the nuances associated with understanding and managing colon polyps. Colon health is a critical aspect of overall well-being, with the colon playing a pivotal role in the digestive system.

As a significant component of the gastrointestinal tract, the colon is responsible for absorbing water and electrolytes, forming and storing feces, and helping the body eliminate waste.

Concerning This Book

In order to empower people with the knowledge to make informed decisions about their digestive health, this comprehensive exploration on conquering colon polyps aims to provide a thorough understanding of the condition, its implications, and effective strategies for prevention and treatment. From risk factors to preventive measures and treatment options, the content within this book is designed to be a valuable resource for both healthcare professionals and individuals seeking to enhance their colon health.

The Significance Of Gut Health

Maintaining optimal colon health is critical because the colon is involved in digestion, nutrient absorption, and waste elimination. A healthy colon also contributes to overall well-being by promoting nutrient absorption, preventing the development of various gastrointestinal disorders, and ensuring proper functioning of the digestive system.

The importance of colon health is further highlighted when one considers the role it plays in preventing conditions like colon polyps, which, if left untreated, can progress to more serious issues like colorectal cancer. Understanding the symbiotic relationship between colon health and overall well-being emphasizes how urgent it is to treat and eradicate colon polyps.

Comprehending Colon Polyps

The term "colon polyps" refers to abnormal growths that develop on the inner lining of the colon or rectum.

These growths can vary in size, shape, and characteristics. While many colon polyps are benign, some may eventually turn cancerous. Knowing the specifics of colon polyps entails learning about risk factors, diagnostic techniques, and the different types of polyps that can appear in the colon. Factors such as age, family history, and certain lifestyle choices can increase the risk of developing colon polyps, so knowing these risk factors is critical for efficient prevention and management. Diagnostic tools like colonoscopies are crucial in identifying and characterizing colon polyps, enabling medical professionals to create treatment plans that are specifically tailored to the individual patient.

Preventive Techniques

Effectively combating colon polyps requires a proactive approach to prevention. Changing one's lifestyle to include eating a diet high in fiber and low in red meat and processed foods can significantly lower the risk of developing colon polyps.

Other important components of a comprehensive prevention strategy include regular physical activity, abstaining from tobacco products, and consuming alcohol in moderation.

Routine screenings, particularly colonoscopies for early detection of polyps, are essential in preventing the progression of benign growths to potentially cancerous entities. Taking preventative action not only lowers the risk of colon polyps but also improves overall colon health, highlighting the holistic approach to conquering this gastrointestinal

Methods Of Treatment

When colon polyps are found, there are a number of different treatment options available, based on the size, type, and location of the polyps. Polypectomy, a common procedure during colonoscopy, involves the removal of polyps and offers benefits for both diagnosis and treatment. More sophisticated methods, such as endoscopic mucosal resection (EMR) and endoscopic submucosal dissection (ESD), may be used for larger polyps or those with particular characteristics. The healthcare provider will often choose the best course of action after carefully evaluating the patient's medical history and the polyps. Patients should engage in discussions with their healthcare providers to understand the reasoning behind the treatment plan that has been selected.

Lifestyle And Nutritional Factors

The role of lifestyle and dietary factors in conquering colon polyps cannot be overstated. Adopting a diet that is high in fiber, fruits, and vegetables while low in red and processed meats has been associated with a reduced risk of developing colon polyps. Fiber, in particular, plays a vital role in promoting regular bowel movements and preventing constipation, which is linked to an increased risk of colon polyps.

Moreover, maintaining a healthy body weight through regular physical activity contributes to overall colon health.

Engaging in regular exercise not only helps in weight management but also reduces inflammation and promotes efficient bowel function. Furthermore, avoiding tobacco products and limiting alcohol consumption are essential lifestyle choices that can contribute to the prevention of colon polyps. By integrating these lifestyle and dietary considerations into daily life, individuals can take proactive steps towards conquering colon polyps and fostering long-term digestive health.

Identifying And Preventing

Screening and early detection are integral components of conquering colon polyps, as they allow for timely intervention and prevention of potential complications. Colonoscopy stands out as a gold standard for colon cancer screening and is a crucial tool for identifying and removing colon polyps. The American Cancer Society recommends regular colonoscopies for individuals aged 45 and older, with earlier screenings for those with a family history of colorectal cancer or other risk factors. Other screening methods, such as fecal occult blood tests (FOBT) and flexible sigmoidoscopy, may also be employed based on individual circumstances.

The effectiveness of these screening methods lies in their ability to detect and characterize colon polyps in their early stages, providing an opportunity for intervention before the polyps progress to malignancy. Emphasizing the importance of regular screenings and early detection is paramount in the overall strategy for conquering colon polyps and reducing the burden of colorectal cancer.

Considering Genetic And Familial Factors

Genetic and familial factors play a significant role in the development of colon polyps. Individuals with a family history of colorectal cancer or a known genetic predisposition, such as familial adenomatous polyposis (FAP) or Lynch syndrome, are at an increased risk of developing colon polyps at an earlier age.

Understanding one's family history and genetic profile is crucial in assessing individual risk and determining appropriate screening protocols. Genetic testing may be recommended for individuals with a family history of hereditary colorectal cancer syndromes to identify specific genetic mutations that increase the risk of polyp formation. In cases where genetic predispositions are identified, personalized screening and management plans can be devised to address the heightened risk and facilitate early detection and intervention.

By integrating genetic and familial considerations into the overall approach to conquering colon polyps, healthcare providers can tailor strategies to the unique needs of individuals with an elevated genetic risk.

Patient Empowerment And Education

Beyond medical interventions, colon polyps can be conquered through patient education and empowerment. Patients can make informed decisions and engage in proactive healthcare by learning about the risk factors, symptoms, and preventive measures associated with colon polyps. Patient empowerment is building a collaborative relationship between patients and healthcare providers that allows for open communication, shared decision-making, and active participation in preventive measures. Patients can take control of their health by becoming more aware of colon health issues, actively participating in screenings, and adopting lifestyle modifications that help prevent colon polyps.

overcoming colon polyps necessitates a multimodal strategy that includes knowing the nuances of colon health, appreciating the value of preventive measures, embracing dietary and lifestyle issues, pushing for routine screenings and early detection, addressing genetic and familial factors, and encouraging patient education and empowerment. By combining these components into a holistic framework, medical professionals and patients can work together to prevent, detect, and treat colon polyps, which will ultimately lessen the incidence of colorectal cancer. Overcoming colon polyps is not just a medical task; it is a shared responsibility that calls for proactive and knowledgeable action from both individuals and healthcare providers.

CHAPTER ONE
COLON POLYPS

Benign growths known as colon polyps, which occur on the inner lining of the colon or rectum and can vary in size and shape, are categorized into three main types: adenomatous polyps, hyperplastic polyps, and inflammatory polyps. Adenomatous polyps are the most common and have the highest risk of progressing to colorectal cancer because they originate from the glandular tissue lining the colon and are therefore considered precancerous.

Hyperplastic polyps, on the other hand, are usually benign and are the product of an overgrowth of normal cells. Finally, inflammatory polyps, as their name implies, appear in response to chronic inflammation of the colon, which is frequently linked to illnesses like Crohn's disease or ulcerative colitis.

Reasons And Danger Elements

The etiology of colon polyps is complex, involving both genetic and environmental factors.

Genetic predisposition is a major risk factor, as people with a family history of colon polyps or colorectal cancer are more susceptible to developing colon polyps. Hereditary conditions like Lynch syndrome and familial adenomatous polyposis (FAP) also increase susceptibility to polyp formation.

Lifestyle choices also play a significant role in the development of colon polyps; diets high in fat, low in fiber, and red and processed meats have been linked to an increased risk. Sedentary behaviors and obesity are also recognized as modifiable risk factors.

Age is another important factor, as the chance of developing colon polyps increases with advancing years.

Signs And Recognition

The fact that colon polyps frequently do not cause any symptoms highlights the value of routine screenings for early detection. When symptoms do appear, they can include rectal bleeding, changes in bowel habits, abdominal pain, and unexplained weight loss. It is important to note that these symptoms can also be indicative of other gastrointestinal conditions, emphasizing the need for a comprehensive diagnostic evaluation.

There are a number of screening techniques used to identify colon polyps, with colonoscopy being the gold standard. Sigmoidoscopy, virtual colonoscopy, and fecal occult blood tests are among the screening options. Each has advantages and disadvantages.

The Value Of Early Identification

Early detection of colon polyps is paramount in preventing the progression to colorectal cancer, one of the leading causes of cancer-related deaths worldwide.

Adenomatous polyps, in particular, have the potential to transform into cancer over time, underscoring the significance of identifying and removing them at an early stage.

Colonoscopy, by allowing for both detection and removal of polyps, serves as a powerful tool for preventing colorectal cancer. The rationale behind early detection lies in the concept of cancer screening as a means of identifying and treating precancerous lesions before they become malignant. Timely intervention not only mitigates the risk of cancer development but also reduces the need for more aggressive treatments and improves overall prognosis. Public awareness campaigns and healthcare initiatives promoting routine screenings play a pivotal role in emphasizing the importance of early detection and encouraging individuals to undergo regular colorectal cancer screenings.

understanding the complexities of colon polyps—their types, causes, symptoms, and the importance of early detection—is critical for efficient prevention and management. By incorporating this understanding into clinical practice and public health initiatives, it is possible to significantly lower the incidence of colorectal cancer and enhance patient outcomes.

CHAPTER TWO
MEDICAL DIAGNOSIS AND TREATMENT

The detection and management of colon polyps are integral components of preventive healthcare, emphasizing early intervention to mitigate the risk of colorectal cancer. Various screening procedures exist to identify colon polyps, with colonoscopy being the gold standard. Colonoscopy involves the insertion of a flexible tube with a camera into the colon, allowing for direct visualization and the removal of polyps during the procedure. This method not only aids in the early detection of polyps but also serves as a therapeutic intervention through polypectomy. Another non-invasive screening option is virtual colonoscopy, utilizing advanced imaging techniques to create a three-dimensional visualization of the colon. While it offers advantages such as reduced invasiveness, it may not be as effective in detecting smaller polyps. Flexible sigmoidoscopy is a procedure that focuses on the lower part of the colon, enabling the visualization and removal of polyps in that region. Other diagnostic tests, such as fecal occult blood tests and stool DNA tests, complement these procedures by identifying blood or genetic markers indicative of polyp presence.

Analyzing Test Findings

After screening is finished, test results must be interpreted in order to determine the course of action to be taken. The results of a colonoscopy are categorized according to the size, number, and histology of the polyps that were found. Adenomatous polyps—particularly those with high-grade dysplasia—are thought to be precursors to colorectal cancer. Hyperplastic polyps—although usually benign—may also be associated with an elevated risk and therefore require close monitoring. The identification of polyps from virtual colonoscopy is categorized according to radiological assessment.

The results of a flexible sigmoidoscopy are assessed in relation to the section of the colon that was visualized during the procedure. Interpretation is a complex process that requires the integration of clinical judgment, patient history, and the results of the test.

Options For Treatment

The treatment of colon polyps involves a number of different approaches, the selection of which is based on variables such as the size, location, and histology of the polyp. Polypectomy, the mainstay of the treatment regimen, is the extraction of polyps from the body during diagnostic procedures such as colonoscopy.

This intervention helps to establish a conclusive diagnosis and also functions as a therapeutic measure, reducing the likelihood of cancer developing. When polyps are large, sessile, or situated in difficult anatomical sites, surgery is required. This method may involve minimally invasive techniques like laparoscopy or traditional open surgery, with the aim of completely removing the polyp. Medications are occasionally taken into consideration for specific types of polyps, particularly when surgery may be necessary.

To sum up, the battle against colon polyps requires a multifaceted strategy that includes screening protocols, careful interpretation of test results, and customized treatment options. Colonoscopy continues to be the most effective screening and intervention tool, offering advantages in both diagnostic and therapeutic domains. Virtual colonoscopy and flexible sigmoidoscopy are two alternative approaches, each with specific benefits and drawbacks. Accurate test result interpretation is critical because it informs subsequent decisions regarding the management of polyps that are detected. Treatment options, such as polypectomy, surgical excision, and, to a lesser extent, medication, take into account the heterogeneous nature of colon polyps and guarantee a patient-centered strategy to reduce the risk of colorectal cancer.

CHAPTER THREE
CHANGES IN LIFESTYLE

The term "colon polyps" refers to abnormal growths that develop in the lining of the colon or rectum. Although most polyps are benign, some may eventually turn cancerous.

Managing and preventing colon polyps requires a multimodal approach, and lifestyle modifications are essential. This section delves into the ideas of physical activity, diet and nutrition, quitting smoking, and reducing alcohol intake as essential elements of a comprehensive strategy to address colon polyps.

Diet and Nutrition: A healthy diet and nutrition are critical in the fight against colon polyps. Eating a balanced, nutrient-dense diet can help lower the chance of developing polyps. Including foods high in fiber, like fruits, vegetables, and whole grains, is important because they not only support regular bowel movements but also offer vital nutrients and antioxidants that fight inflammation and oxidative stress, two factors that are linked to the formation of colon polyps.

Foods to Include: A diet high in cruciferous vegetables, such as broccoli, cauliflower, and Brussels sprouts, has been shown to be effective in lowering the incidence of colon polyps.

These vegetables contain bioactive compounds, such as sulforaphane, which have been shown to have anti-carcinogenic properties.

High-antioxidant fruits, such as berries, can also have a protective effect against polyps. Whole grains, legumes, and lean proteins, like fish, poultry, and beans, should also be essential parts of a diet designed to prevent colon polyps.

Eats to Avoid: There are certain dietary choices that can increase the risk of colon polyps, and knowing these factors is important for effective prevention. Red and processed meats have been linked to a higher risk of colorectal cancer, so consuming them in moderation is advised.

High intake of saturated and trans fats, which are frequently found in fried and processed foods, should be reduced. Finally, cutting back on sugary drinks and snacks can help you maintain a healthier diet and prevent colon polyps.

Exercise: There is a strong correlation between regular physical activity and a lower risk of both colorectal cancer and colon polyps. Moderate-intensity exercises, like brisk walking, cycling, or swimming, can provide protective effects for at least 150 minutes per week. Exercise has been shown to help regulate bowel movements, reduce inflammation, and strengthen the immune system—all of which are critical in preventing the development of colon polyps. Additionally, maintaining a healthy weight through regular physical activity is linked to a lower risk of colorectal cancer, emphasizing the importance of exercise in combating colon polyps.

Smoking Cessation: Cigarette smoke contains a variety of carcinogens that can negatively affect the cells lining the colon and rectum, increasing the likelihood of polyp formation.

Cessation not only lowers the risk of polyp formation but also has numerous other health benefits. One of the most important ways to combat colon polyps is to quit smoking.

The earlier a person quits, the greater the reduction in colorectal cancer risk, highlighting the urgency of addressing this modifiable risk factor.

Reducing Alcohol Consumption: Drinking too much alcohol has been associated with a higher risk of colorectal cancer. As a result, reducing alcohol consumption is essential to beating colon polyps. The mechanisms through which alcohol causes colorectal cancer are complicated and may include the conversion of alcohol into acetaldehyde, a known carcinogen, as well as its effects on the absorption of folate and DNA synthesis. To reduce these risks, it is recommended that alcohol be consumed in accordance with recommended guidelines, such as one drink for women and two for men.

In summary, lifestyle changes are critical to the battle against colon polyps. Diet and nutrition, exercise, quitting smoking, and consuming less alcohol are all important lifestyle modifications that not only help prevent colon polyps but also improve overall health and well-being. Taking a comprehensive approach that includes these lifestyle changes can help people take charge of their health and reduce their risk of colon polyps and, consequently, colorectal cancer.

CHAPTER FOUR

MANAGING STRESS AND MENTAL HEALTH

An individual's overall well-being is greatly influenced by stress, which has been shown to have a negative impact on colon health.

Prolonged stress has been linked to a number of physiological changes in the body, and new research indicates that stress may also be linked to the formation of colon polyps. Stress causes the release of hormones like cortisol, which when persistently elevated, can lead to inflammation and altered immune responses in the colon. This chronic low-grade inflammation may create an environment that is favorable to the formation of polyps, which are precursors to colorectal cancer. It is crucial to comprehend the complex relationship between stress and colon health in order to develop comprehensive strategies for managing and preventing colon polyps.

Coping Mechanisms

Individuals can use a variety of coping strategies to address the relationship between stress and colon polyps in an effective manner. One important way to manage stress is to incorporate relaxation techniques into daily routines.

These techniques, such as progressive muscle relaxation and deep breathing exercises, help reduce tension and the physiological response to stress. Additionally, mindfulness and meditation practices are powerful tools for building mental resilience. Mindfulness entails paying deliberate attention to the present moment, while meditation promotes a state of deep relaxation and heightened awareness. By integrating these practices, individuals can create a buffer against stress.

Techniques For Relaxation

Relaxation techniques comprise a range of approaches intended to elicit a state of tranquility and diminish the physiological arousal linked to stress. Controlled breathing exercises, for example, concentrate on deliberate inhalation and exhalation patterns, fostering relaxation and lessening the influence of the body's stress reaction. Progressive muscle relaxation progresses by gradually tensing and then relaxing various muscle groups, contributing to the reduction of overall tension. Visualization techniques, in which people mentally transport themselves to a calm and serene setting, can augment the effectiveness of relaxation practices. Frequent application of these techniques into daily life not only reduces stress but also plays a pivotal role in the prevention and management of

Meditation And Mindfulness

The integration of mindfulness and meditation into daily life not only helps reduce stress but may also prevent colon polyps. Mindfulness is the cultivation of an elevated awareness of the present moment without judgment. It is a practice that encourages people to observe their thoughts and emotions objectively, fostering a resilient mental state.

On the other hand, meditation is a broad category that includes practices like transcendental meditation, loving-kindness meditation, and mindfulness meditation. These approaches have been shown to modulate the body's stress response, lowering cortisol levels and promoting a sense of well-being.

Assistive Systems

Building strong support networks is essential to managing stress effectively and, as a result, preventing colon polyps. Social support from friends, family, and the community is crucial to reducing the negative effects of stressors on mental health. Having a trustworthy network of people who can provide emotional support, encouragement, and understanding can greatly increase stress resilience. Support groups and therapy sessions also offer a structured setting in which people can share experiences and coping mechanisms.

The group's sharing of successes and challenges creates a sense of community and reinforces healthy coping strategies. By cultivating strong support networks, people can improve their capacity to manage stress and prevent colon polyps.

the relationship between stress and colon health is intricate and multifaceted, and it requires attention when it comes to preventing colon polyps. Reducing stress with the help of mindfulness, meditation, relaxation techniques, and strong support networks is a comprehensive strategy for protecting both mental health and colon health. Through comprehension and application of these coping mechanisms, people can empower themselves to deal with the difficulties of contemporary life while encouraging a lifestyle that is healthy for their colons.

CHAPTER FIVE
PREVENTION STRATEGIES

It is impossible to overstate the significance of routine check-ups when it comes to eliminating colon polyps. Medical examinations, such as colonoscopies and other screening procedures, are essential for the early detection and prevention of colon polyps. Regular examinations allow medical professionals to recognize and track any abnormal growths or polyps in the colon, allowing for prompt intervention and treatment.

People are strongly encouraged to have regular screenings, particularly if they have a family history of colorectal issues or other risk factors.

Early detection reduces the likelihood that polyps will become more serious conditions, like colorectal cancer.

Another critical component of treating colon polyps is surveillance after polyp removal.

Because polyps can recur even after they are successfully removed, surveillance involves routine follow-up screenings to keep an eye out for any indications of new polyp formation.

Vigilance after treatment is necessary to identify and promptly address any potential problems.

Medical professionals may suggest a customized surveillance schedule based on the number and type of polyps removed, the patient's overall health, and their family history. This continuous monitoring is essential to preventing polyp recurrence and lowering the risk of colorectal cancer development.

In order to effectively combat colon polyps, both genetic counseling and screening are essential. While some people are genetically predisposed to developing polyps or colorectal cancer, genetic counseling helps people understand their familial risk factors and provides insights into the likelihood of developing colon polyps; this information is useful in customizing screening and prevention strategies.

Genetic screening, on the other hand, involves analyzing an individual's DNA for specific markers associated with colorectal conditions and further improves the precision of preventive measures.

An effective campaign to combat colon polyps must focus on public education and awareness because well-informed people are more likely to adopt preventive measures,

get regular screenings, and make lifestyle decisions that lower the risk of polyp formation. Public awareness campaigns should educate the public about the significance of early detection, risk factors, and preventive strategies.

Educational initiatives can target a variety of demographic groups by highlighting the importance of a healthy lifestyle, balanced diet, and regular exercise in preventing colon polyps. Additionally, increasing awareness about the availability and accessibility of screening programs can motivate more people to take proactive steps to preventive healthcare, which will improve overall health.

the complex strategy for eliminating colon polyps includes a variety of preventive techniques. Routine examinations lay the groundwork for early detection, and surveillance following polyp removal guarantees ongoing observation and intervention. Genetic counseling and screening give a customized aspect to preventive measures by addressing individual risk factors.

Public awareness and education act as a stimulant for the widespread adoption of preventive practices. By addressing these preventive techniques in their entirety, the medical community can achieve notable progress in lowering the incidence and impact of colon polyps.

of colon polyps, eventually contributing to the more general objective of averting colorectal cancer.

The key to preventing colon polyps is routine medical examinations, which are essential for the early identification of any abnormalities in the colon, including the presence of polyps.

The importance of routine medical examinations is that they can detect potential problems early on, when they are easier to manage.

People are strongly advised to have periodic screenings, especially if they have risk factors, such as a family history of colorectal diseases or other conditions that predispose them to the condition. Early detection not only increases the chance of a successful treatment, but it also reduces the risk of polyps developing into more serious conditions like colorectal cancer.

A crucial part of eliminating colon polyps is surveillance after polyps are removed.

The removal of polyps does not ensure that they will never recur, so monitoring the colon after treatment is necessary. This continuous watch is intended to identify any new polyp formation as soon as possible. Medical professionals can customize surveillance plans according to the type and quantity of polyps removed, the patient's general health, and their family history. By closely monitoring the colon, the medical community hopes to avoid polyp recurrence and reduce the likelihood of colorectal cancer development.

A customized element is added to the overall plan for overcoming colon polyps through genetic counseling and screening. Certain people have a genetic predisposition to either polyps or colorectal cancer, and genetic counseling is essential in identifying these familial risk factors.

It also provides individuals with knowledge about their genetic composition, which helps to personalize screening and prevention plans. Genetic screening, which involves testing a person's DNA for specific markers linked to colorectal conditions, improves the accuracy of preventive measures. The identification of genetic predispositions allows medical practitioners to develop customized plans for surveillance and early intervention, which greatly contributes to the prevention of colon polyps.

Public awareness and education stand as fundamental pillars in the collective effort to conquer colon polyps. An informed and educated population is more likely to adopt preventive measures, including regular screenings and lifestyle choices that minimize the risk of polyp formation. Public awareness campaigns should disseminate information about the critical aspects of early detection, risk factors, and preventive strategies. Educational initiatives can be tailored to different demographics, emphasizing the significance of a healthy lifestyle, a balanced diet, and regular exercise in preventing colon polyps. Moreover, raising awareness about the availability and accessibility of screening programs is essential to encourage more individuals to proactively engage in preventive healthcare measures. Ultimately, a well-informed public is crucial to the success of conquering colon polyps, as it fosters a proactive approach to healthcare and empowers individuals to take charge of their well-being.

a thorough and multifaceted approach to eliminating colon polyps includes a variety of preventive strategies, each of which contributes in a different way to the overall goal of preventing colorectal cancer. For example, routine check-ups establish early detection, surveillance following polyp removal guarantees continuous monitoring, and genetic counseling/screening provides individualized insights into individual risk factors. Public awareness and education also act as catalysts for the widespread adoption of preventive practices, which together significantly reduce the incidence and impact of colon polyps. As a result, the medical community can make significant progress toward the ultimate goal of eliminating colon polyps.

CHAPTER SIX
TRUE NARRATIVES
Experiences Of Patients

It is critical for researchers and healthcare professionals to comprehend patient experiences in the context of overcoming colon polyps.

Patients undergoing screening, diagnosis, and treatment for colon polyps navigate a complex healthcare environment involving a variety of medical procedures and interventions.

Receiving a colon polyp diagnosis has significant psychological and emotional ramifications; patients frequently experience fear, anxiety, and uncertainty as they consider the implications of their diagnosis and the possibility that it will progress to colorectal cancer.

The patient experience is a range of feelings that patients may experience, starting from the screening phase when they may be anxious about the process and ending with the post-treatment phase when they may feel relieved or worried about the possibility of polyps returning. Additionally, the support and communication that patients receive from healthcare providers is a significant factor in the patient experience. Empathetic and transparent communication can reduce anxiety and build trust between patients and healthcare providers.

In addition, patient experiences differ according to age, gender, and socioeconomic status.

Patients who are older may have different difficulties managing their colon polyps than patients who are younger. Patients' perceptions and management strategies may also be influenced by their access to healthcare resources and information. It is critical to analyze and comprehend these varied experiences in order to create patient-centered strategies for effectively treating colon polyps.

Success Narratives

Stories of individuals who have successfully undergone screening, received prompt diagnosis, and received effective treatment—all of which have resulted in the eradication or successful management of colon polyps—serve as rays of hope and inspiration for patients and healthcare providers alike. They also highlight the significance of early detection and intervention, highlighting the positive outcomes that can be achieved through proactive healthcare measures.

Success stories can be used as educational tools, providing insights into best practices, cutting-edge treatments, and strategies for preventing the recurrence of colon polyps. They also further illuminate the role of multidisciplinary healthcare teams by highlighting examples of collaboration between gastroenterologists, surgeons, oncologists, and other specialists that have led to successful patient outcomes. Lastly, they contribute to the dissemination of knowledge within the medical community and empower patients to actively participate in their healthcare journey.

Though individual responses to treatment may differ depending on a number of factors, including the patient's general health, the effectiveness of the chosen intervention, and the stage at which the polyp developed, it is important to acknowledge that success stories may not be universal. Nevertheless, by looking at success stories, medical professionals can spot trends, improve treatment plans, and continuously raise the standard of care for patients with colon polyps.

Obstacles and Achievements

Overcoming colon polyps is not without its difficulties, and knowing the setbacks as well as the successes in this process is critical for all-encompassing healthcare plans. Difficulties occur at different phases, from the initial screening and diagnosis to the treatment of recurring polyps or the possible development of colorectal cancer. One major difficulty is spreading awareness regarding the significance of routine screenings and early detection, since many people may be afraid, misinformed, or unaware of the need for screening procedures.

On the other hand, successes come from the successful implementation of comprehensive screening programs by healthcare systems, which allow for the early detection and removal of polyps. Addressing healthcare disparities is another aspect of overcoming challenges, since certain populations may encounter obstacles that prevent them from receiving timely screenings or appropriate treatments. Success comes from healthcare initiatives that prioritize inclusivity and strive to eliminate these disparities.

Success stories of individual patients are just one aspect of the victory over colon polyps; systemic improvements in healthcare delivery, public awareness, and medical research are all important. Additionally, innovations in endoscopic techniques, imaging modalities, and treatment options improve the precision and efficacy of interventions.

Collaborative research efforts offer valuable insights into the genetic and molecular aspects of colon polyps, paving the way for personalized treatment approaches.

Finally, a thorough understanding of how to overcome colon polyps is derived from a combination of patient experiences, success stories, challenges, and triumphs. By investigating these ideas, medical professionals can improve their methods, create patient-centered strategies, and further the field's progress. By recognizing the emotional and physical aspects of the patient experience, taking note of successful outcomes, resolving obstacles, and commemorating victories, the medical community can cooperate to improve colon polyp prevention, early detection, and management.

CHAPTER SEVEN
FUTURE TRENDS AND RESEARCH
New Technologies

In the field of colon polyp management, emerging technologies are essential for both diagnosis and treatment. One significant development is the application of artificial intelligence (AI) to medical imaging for polyp detection. Machine learning algorithms are capable of accurately analyzing colonoscopy images, which helps clinicians identify and characterize polyps more precisely. This enhances screening processes overall and improves diagnostic capabilities.

Furthermore, the development of advanced endoscopic technologies has demonstrated promise in the identification and removal of colon polyps. For example, high-definition and high-magnification endoscopes offer a clearer view of the mucosal surface of the colon, which enables a more accurate identification of subtle polyps. Additionally, robotic-assisted colonoscopy systems are becoming more popular, providing enhanced maneuverability and stability during procedures.

These technologies not only reduce procedural risks but also improve polyp detection efficaciously.

The genetic basis of colon polyps is also being better understood thanks to genomic technologies. Advances in genetic sequencing and analysis have made it possible to identify specific genetic mutations linked to the development of polyps, which helps identify individuals who are at higher risk early on and provides opportunities for targeted therapies based on the genetic characteristics of the polyps.

Improvements In Medical Care

Endoscopic mucosal resection (EMR) and endoscopic submucosal dissection (ESD) are now standard procedures for removing larger polyps without invasive surgery because they allow for precise removal and histological examination, which ensures complete eradication of the polyp while minimizing the impact on surrounding tissues. Significant advancements in colon polyp treatment have resulted in more personalized and effective therapeutic strategies.

In addition, the development of minimally invasive surgical methods, like laparoscopic and robotic-assisted surgeries, has revolutionized the way complex cases are managed.

These methods provide better cosmetic results, quicker recovery from open surgery, and less pain after surgery. These improvements also improve patient experiences and treatment compliance.

Clinical trials investigating the efficacy of immunotherapy in combination with conventional treatments are underway, paving the way for more comprehensive and effective therapeutic approaches. Immunotherapy has emerged as a promising avenue for the treatment of advanced colon polyps and colorectal cancer. Immunotherapeutic agents show potential in preventing polyp recurrence and inhibiting cancer progression by targeting and eliminating abnormal cells with the help of the body's immune system.

Prospective Fields Of Study

Research on colon polyps is still ongoing in a variety of areas with the goal of improving current practices and pursuing new directions in both prevention and treatment. An increasing amount of attention has been paid to the microbiome's role in colorectal health, with studies examining the impact of gut bacteria on the development and progression of polyps. By comprehending the complex interactions between the microbiome and the host, new preventive measures and therapeutic targets may become apparent.

In addition, research into the role of lifestyle factors, such as diet and physical activity, in modulating colorectal health is ongoing and offers insights into population-level preventive measures. Epigenetic research holds promise in elucidating the molecular mechanisms underlying colon polyp formation. When epigenetic modifications associated with polyps are identified, targeted therapies aimed at reversing or mitigating these alterations may be developed.

Nanoparticles engineered to target specific molecular markers associated with polyps can improve the accuracy of diagnostic procedures and deliver therapeutic agents directly to the affected tissue, minimizing side effects and improving treatment efficacy.

This targeted approach presents a promising frontier in colon polyp research. Nanotechnology advancements offer novel approaches for drug delivery and imaging in colon polyp management.

CONCLUSION

technological advancements, treatment modalities, and ongoing research endeavors are transforming the landscape of colon polyp management. Artificial intelligence is being incorporated into diagnostic processes, endoscopic techniques are being refined, and genomic and immunotherapeutic approaches are emerging, which are changing the way we detect and treat colon polyps. As we continue to explore promising research areas like the microbiome, epigenetics, and nanotechnology, we hope to gain a more nuanced understanding of the factors influencing polyp development and progression.

Together, these advancements are leading to a paradigm shift in colon polyp management toward more individualized and targeted approaches. Future developments promise improved screening, accurate diagnosis, and customized therapeutic interventions, which will ultimately improve patient outcomes and lessen the global burden of colorectal diseases. As the complexity of colon polyps continues to be uncovered, cooperation between clinicians, researchers, and technology developers will be critical to bringing these advances from the lab to the clinic and ushering in a new era in colorectal health.